CANCER
and the
WORKER

'Tis a sordid profit that's accompanied
by the destruction of Health.
—Bernardino Ramazzini
Treatise on the Diseases of
Tradesmen (1705)

The New York Academy of Sciences
New York, New York
1977

Second printing, March, 1978.

Library of Congress Cataloging in Publication Data

Lehmann, Phyllis.
    Cancer and the worker.

    "Based on volume 271 of the Annals, entitled
Occupational carcinogenesis."
       1. Carcinogens. 2. Cancer—Prevention.
3. Occupational diseases. I. Occupational
carcinogenesis. II. Title.
RC268.6.L43   616.9'94'071   77-25215
ISBN 0-89072-058-4

The New York Academy of Sciences believes that it has a responsibility to
encourage the dissemination of scientific information. For this reason, Volume
271, *Occupational Carcinogenesis,* has been rewritten for the general public.
Every attempt has been made to produce a scientifically accurate work, but in
the process of abridgement scientific detail will inevitably be lost. Positions
taken by the participants in the conference from whose reports this volume
derives are their own and not those of The Academy. The Academy has no
intent to influence legislation by the publishing of such opinions.

PCP
Printed in the United States of America
ISBN 0-89072-058-4

Contents

Acknowledgments

This book is based on Volume 271 of the Annals, entitled *Occupational Carcinogenesis,* published by The New York Academy of Sciences in May of 1976. *Occupational Carcinogenesis* consisted of a collection of papers presented at a conference of the same name, held in March of 1975. That conference was chaired by Dr. Umberto Saffiotti of the National Cancer Institute and by Dr. Joseph K. Wagoner of the National Institute for Occupational Safety and Health. The conference was sponsored by The New York Academy of Sciences, Group Health Incorporated, the National Cancer Institute, the National Institute for Occupational Safety and Health, and the Society for Occupational and Environmental Health.

The idea for a book to be written to and for workers was voiced by Dr. Sidney Wolfe of the Citizen's Health Research Group. The adaptation was written by Ms. Phyllis Lehmann. Various persons reviewed the original manuscript and made valuable suggestions. Chief among them were Dr. Umberto Saffiotti, Dr. Irving J. Selikoff, Dr. Joseph K. Wagoner, and Mr. Sheldon W. Samuels. Financial support for the writing of this book was provided by the National Institute for Occupational Safety and Health.

Bill M. Boland
Executive Editor

List of Cancer Terms

Cancer—a general term for a large group of diseases characterized by the uncontrolled growth and spread of abnormal cells. Cancer is the Latin word for crab.

Carcinoma—the most common malignant tumor.

Leukemia—a disease in which abnormal leukocytes (white blood cells) accumulate in the blood and bone marrow.

Lymphoma—a disease in which abnormal numbers of lymphocytes (a type of leukocyte) are produced by the spleen and lymph nodes.

Sarcoma—a malignant tumor of certain tissues, such as muscle or bone.

Cancer-causing substances—people are probably exposed to many carcinogens in small amounts, rather than to large doses of a single carcinogen, such as are used in animal tests. Accumulation of the effects of these small doses—sometimes added to by relatively large doses of carcinogens as in the workplace—leads to cancer. It is often not possible to say that a particular carcinogen causes cancer. Instead, we say that exposure to a carcinogen increases the risk of developing cancer. The higher the exposure, the greater the risk.

Carcinogen—anything that produces cancer when it comes into contact with animals or humans by any route of exposure (such as the lungs, skin, or gastrointestinal tract).

Malignant—leading toward progressive invasion of body tissues and probably ending in death. Generally, the tumor invades nearby tissue and spreads to other parts of the body.

Mutagen—anything that causes a mutation. Most carcinogens are also mutagens. Testing a substance to see if it is a mutagen may turn out to be a fairly reliable way to tell if it is a carcinogen. Such tests are easier, faster, and cheaper than the usual animal tests, since they can be done with bacteria.

Mutation—a change in genetic make-up that can be passed from generation to generation.

Occupational cancer—cancer caused by carcinogens present in the work environment or encountered during performance of the job.

Tumor—an abnormal growth that grows faster than normal tissue and that may continue to grow even after the original cause is removed.

Part I
INTRODUCTION

"Cancer" is one of the most frightening words in our language. And with good reason. This year 675,000 Americans will find out they have it. Some 370,000 will die of it—one every one-and-a-half minutes.

At present rates, one in four Americans now living will eventually have cancer. It can be expected to strike in two of every three families.

True, there has been some progress. About 1.5 million former cancer patients are alive, cured of the disease. Yet, of every six people who get cancer today, two will be saved and four will die.

And the cancer rates have been going up steadily. In 1973, 351,000 Americans died of cancer; in 1974, 357,000; in 1975, 364,000. Why the increase? Some of the increase is due to the aging of our people. But some we can't easily explain.

The World Health Organization estimates that between 75 and 85 percent of all cancers are caused by environmental exposures. Certainly, some (many?) of those exposures take place on the job, and others are the result of the spread of the same agents into the community at large.

No one knows for sure just how many workers are exposed to cancer-causing substances, known as *carcinogens*, because no one is certain just how many different chemicals are in use today, or how many of them can cause cancer. The National Institute for Occupational Safety and Health (NIOSH) lists

1

1,500 substances that have shown some evidence of causing cancer. But neither NIOSH scientists nor anyone else knows how many of these can be found in the workplace or what dangers they pose for workers. If we consider only the carcinogens that are *known* to be present in various workplaces, however, over six million workers are now being exposed to them! If we include all past exposures as well as the current ones, the number is astounding (over one million for asbestos alone).

We suspect that chemical mixtures as diverse as coke-oven emissions and some anesthetic gases used in hospital operating rooms can cause cancer. We know that asbestos, arsenic, and vinyl chloride, to name a few of the well-known villains, can cause cancer. We *do* have data on many of the hazards workers are exposed to, but we *don't* know how many more "vinyl chlorides" are out there. (We didn't know about vinyl chloride until 1974.) We *do* know that cancer is one of the most serious occupational health problems in the United States today. We *don't* know how to convince society to make the hard decisions necessary to control it.

This book is designed to inform you—the worker, the plant manager, the union leader—about what we do and don't know about occupational cancer and about the issues involved in its control.

Chapter 1
The Bicentennial
We Don't Celebrate

Amid the Bicentennial hoopla of the past few years, another 200th anniversary came and went. It's one we aren't too proud of—the bicentennial of the discovery of occupational cancer.

In 1775 Percivall Pott, an English surgeon, reported finding cancer of the scrotum among London chimney sweeps. On their jobs, these chimney sweeps had been exposed, as children in the grimy soot, to the by-products of coal combustion, which we now know can cause cancer. The sad fact is that during the 200 years following Pott's discovery, our record in protecting workers from cancer has been poor. For example:

- Thousands of coke-oven workers in the steel industry are still inhaling the same kinds of substances that caused cancer among the chimney sweeps. The result: they are dying of lung cancer at a rate 10 times that of other steelworkers.

- One hundred years ago miners in Central Europe were found to be dying of lung cancer. Fifty years ago, scientists identified radioactivity in the mines as the cause of their disease. Yet in 1971, thousands of American uranium miners were working with radioactive materials under conditions that tripled their chances of dying from lung cancer.

- Today, 130 years after scrotal cancer was discovered among copper smelters exposed to arsenic, some 1.5 million American workers are inhaling the same substance. They're also dying

3

of lung and lymphatic cancer at two to eight times the average national rate.

- Eighty years ago scientists discovered that aromatic amines were causing bladder cancer among German dye workers. Such amines as benzidine and beta-naphthylamine were banned or taken off the market decades ago in the United Kingdom, Switzerland, Japan, Italy, and the Soviet Union.* Yet in 1973, thousands of American workers were still literally sloshing around in these chemicals. These workers are now developing—and will continue to develop—bladder tumors at an epidemic rate. As of three years ago, half (27) of the former employees at one benzidine plant had developed bladder cancer.

- Seventy-five years ago asbestos was known to cause a fatal lung disease. It was identified 25 years ago as a potent cause of lung cancer. But very recently, workers in dozens of asbestos factories and hundreds of asbestos-related trades were laboring in asbestos dust so thick that it blocked the light. The grim outlook: of 1 million current and former asbestos workers in this country, 300,000–400,000 can expect to die of cancer, more than double the national rate.

The long reach of cancer

The cancer epidemic is all the more tragic because it doesn't stop at the factory gates. Look at asbestos. Wives, children, and other relatives of many asbestos workers have died of cancer—and more will die—because they were exposed to asbestos carried home on work clothes and shoes. People who live close to asbestos factories have also developed cancer. And nearly all city dwellers on whom autopsies are performed have some asbestos in their lungs.

Look at arsenic. People living in areas sprayed with arsenic pesticides are dying of lung cancer at an increased rate. Children living near copper smelters have unusually high levels of arsenic in their hair and urine.

We now know that asbestos and arsenic, as well as count-

---

* There is uncertainty, however, about how well these restrictions have been observed.

less other carcinogens, are present in our water because of industry's uncontrolled disposal of wastes.

Perhaps the most chilling example of what workers and society may face in the future is vinyl chloride. For 35 years this gas has been a key ingredient in the manufacture of plastics. It wasn't until 1974, however, that we learned it was a potent cause of liver cancer. Several hundred thousand workers may be exposed to vinyl chloride on the job. But no one knows how many tens of thousands of people are exposed to it because they live near a plant where vinyl chloride or polyvinyl chloride is made. No one knows how many hundreds of thousands of people have been exposed because they used aerosol sprays in which vinyl chloride was used as a propellant and solvent. And, no one knows what the consequences of these exposures will be. Of course, there may be no consequences. We just don't know.

A "social disease"

If society doesn't take the steps necessary to control environmental cancer, we may face an increasing, and perhaps irreversible, public health hazard. Each year industry begins using hundreds of new chemicals whose potential for causing cancer has never been tested. One hope for stemming this chemical tide is the Toxic Substances Control Act, passed by Congress in September of 1976. This law gives the government authority to require testing of possibly hazardous substances *before* they go on the market.

The solution, though, doesn't rest just with the politicians or the scientists. Cancer is everybody's problem. It is a social disease whose causes and control are deeply rooted in our technology. A large percentage of cancers can be prevented, but doing so will require effort from all parts of society.

Chapter 2
A Unique Disease

What is cancer?

"Cancer" has been defined as a large group of diseases characterized by the uncontrolled growth and spread of abnormal cells. If this spread continues, the victim dies.

Usually when a foreign substance causes toxic or other undesirable changes in the body, the damaged cells either heal or eventually die and are replaced by scar tissue or by normal cells. Cancer is unique because the affected cells continue to multiply and produce new abnormal cells even after the body is no longer exposed to the original cancer-causing substance.

What causes cancer?

If scientists really knew the answer to that question you probably wouldn't be reading this book, because there would most likely be ways to prevent this most dreaded disease. No one knows just what causes cancer to develop, but we are pretty certain that a number of factors contribute to its development. Many scientists suspect that there is no cancer without a carcinogen and it is thought that there is seldom just one carcinogen. A person's genetic make-up, habits, cultural background, and general health status all help to determine whether or not he/she will develop cancer, and if so, how rapidly it will spread.

Among the factors that seem to influence the development of cancer are:

- **Enzymes.** Susceptibility to certain kinds of cancer may depend on the activities of various enzymes, which are proteins that influence chemical reactions in the body.
- **The body's immune defense system.**
- **Hormones.**
- **Smoking.** Smoking is known to cause lung and other cancers.
- **Diet.** According to one theory, eating smoked foods, for example, can increase the risk of cancer, whereas such metals as zinc in the diet can decrease the risk.
- **Air pollution.**
- **Exposure to industrial chemicals.**
- **Use of medications.** In our drug-oriented society, scientists suspect this could sometimes be a factor.
- **Infection with viruses or bacteria.**
- **Age.** The risk of cancer is greatest at two periods during our life spans—childhood and old age. Of growing concern is the possibility that a child may develop cancer as the result of his/her mother's on-the-job exposure to cancer-causing substances during pregnancy. Many substances, including carcinogens, easily pass through the placenta from the mother's bloodstream into the blood of the unborn child. This danger is becoming more significant as more women enter the labor force in a wider variety of industrial jobs. On one coke-oven battery, for example, 20 percent of the employees are now women.

Doctors have long recognized that occupational cancer was not simply the result of exposure to a carcinogen. In the early 1900s, researchers noted that a person's genetic characteristics, such as skin pigmentation, helped determine whether he/she would develop skin cancer after exposure to ultraviolet light. Another scientist reporting on skin cancers among Scottish oil shale workers observed that some workers had a greater tendency to develop cancer than did others, even though working conditions were the same for all. The first experimental evidence of this so-called multiple-factor effect came in 1927 when two researchers showed that skin cancer in laboratory animals was more likely to develop if the skin was scratched before coming into contact with tar.

Exposure to combinations of chemicals at the same time can also affect cancer development. Unfortunately, most laboratory studies are done on one chemical at a time; but in the real workplace people are almost never exposed to just a single carcinogen.

There is evidence that some substances acting together will cause more tumors within a shorter period of time than either one acting separately. Scientists call such substances *co-carcinogens.* The rates of cancer among asbestos workers and uranium miners who smoke are much higher than the rates among those who do not smoke, probably as a result of such combined action. In laboratory animal experiments, two carcinogens, benzpyrene and a nitrosamine, produced few or no tumors when given separately, but combined administration of the two gave rise to a high incidence of tumors.

In some cases, a substance that does not cause cancer itself will serve as a co-carcinogen, prodding a carcinogen into action. In studies done in the 1940s, researchers applied a cancer-causing substance to the skin of experimental animals. Scarcely any cancers appeared. But when the carcinogen was followed by a dose of a noncarcinogenic substance, in this case croton oil, tumors developed in almost all the animals. The croton oil seemed to be "promoting" the effect of the carcinogen. Since that time, scientists have discovered a number of chemicals shown to be capable of promoting the effects of carcinogens.

Is cancer reversible?

At very early stages, abnormal cell growth may be reversible, but later it becomes irreversible and finally malignant—spreading throughout the affected organ and then to other parts of the body. Environmental factors can not only trigger abnormal cell growth; they can also determine whether a new cell growth becomes malignant.

Most scientists agree that cancer is basically an irreversible process because the affected cells continue to multiply even after exposure to a carcinogen has stopped.

There is dramatic evidence that the effects of exposure to

some cancer-causing substances are irreversible. For example, short exposures to benzidine have caused tumors 30 years after exposure ended. Brief exposure to asbestos has caused cancer decades later. Vinyl chloride has been found in the bodies of heavily exposed workers as long as five years after their last exposure. A number of other carcinogens—such as dieldrin, DDT, PCBs, ethylene dichloride, ethylene dibromide, and beryllium—also persist in body tissues for long periods. Once the exposure has taken place, the potential for cancer apparently remains indefinitely.

How much exposure to a carcinogen does it take to cause cancer?

No one really knows. Some scientists, including a number who work for industry, argue that the amount, or dose, of a carcinogen is significant. As evidence they point to studies of certain high-risk groups of workers who were exposed to the same chemical. Only a certain percentage developed cancer, and generally those who did develop it were the ones who had the highest exposures. This indicates, these scientists say, that there may be a "threshold" limit of exposure, below which a carcinogen will not cause cancer.

However, most occupational cancer experts believe that there is *no* safe exposure to a cancer-causing substance. And they have solid arguments to back them up. As mentioned above, even short exposures to a carcinogen can cause cancer many years later. This delay from time of exposure to the time disease develops is called the *latent period*. For occupational cancer, it ranges from 10 to 50 or more years, but averages more than 20. In some cases, such as skin cancer caused by exposure to coal tar pitch, the latent period may be as short as two years.

Dr. Irving J. Selikoff of New York City's Mount Sinai School of Medicine cites a study of 250 asbestos workers exposed at least 25 years ago to heavy concentrations of asbestos for three months or less. Even though their exposures were brief, these workers still died of lung cancer at three-and-a-half times the expected rate. It is conceivable that a worker could be heavily exposed to asbestos for just one day and develop cancer years later as a result of that exposure. He may have worked with asbestos for only one day, but his lungs continue to be exposed to the asbestos deposits trapped there.

Because of the long latent period for most carcinogens, even the effects of brief or low-level exposures on today's workers won't be known for several more decades. Simply waiting to see what happens is playing Russian roulette with workers' lives. Therefore, most scientists believe that the only sure way to prevent occupational cancer is to prevent exposure to carcinogens in the first place.

This is especially important since even early diagnosis of some cancers, such as lung cancer, doesn't improve the survival rate. For example, scientists from Mount Sinai carefully observed 1,249 New York City area asbestos insulation workers from 1963 through 1974. Out of this group, 59 workers—mostly those who had begun working with asbestos 20 or more years previously—developed lung cancer. Even though each worker had been regularly examined and x-rayed and their cancers detected early, 57 out of the 59 died. Obviously, better methods for earlier diagnosis and treatment of cancer are needed. But in the meantime, the only real solution to occupational cancer is to clean up the workplace.

How many chemicals cause cancer?

No one knows. The National Institute for Occupational Safety and Health (NIOSH) lists some 1,500 substances that have shown some evidence of being associated with neoplasms —that is, tumors or abnormal growths.

Approximately one in every 10 substances now being added to NIOSH's mammoth Toxic Substances List is a carcinogen. But again, there is no way of knowing how many of these are commonly present in the workplace, although it is safe to assume that most of them are present at one time or another—as products, by-products, waste products, or uninvited contaminants.

In order to establish priorities for regulating these carcinogens, NIOSH is trying to find out more about them: How much of each chemical is produced each year? How much is imported? What industries use it? How is it used and how are workers exposed to it? How many people are handling it? Are there substitutes available that would work just as well? Have there been any human cancers that can be linked with exposure to it?

NIOSH is also constantly on the lookout for other chemicals not yet on its carcinogens list that might be related to an unusual number of cancer deaths among certain groups of workers.

With support from the National Cancer Institute, the International Agency for Research on Cancer (IARC), in Lyon, France, has been preparing reports on specific chemicals that are suspected of causing cancer in humans. The eight volumes completed so far cover 196 chemicals.* Of these, 17 have shown evidence of causing cancer in man. In most cases, proof was established by studying workers who were exposed to these chemicals on the job.

The Agency's list includes many familiar industrial hazards, such as asbestos, arsenic compounds, 4-aminobiphenyl, auramine, benzene, benzidine, bis(chloromethyl)ether, cadmium oxide and sulphate, chromium, hematite, 2-naphthylamine, nickel, soot and tars, and vinyl chloride. See page 12.

Of the 196 chemicals evaluated in the first eight volumes of the IARC Monograph series, there is unquestionable evidence that 94 cause cancer in animals. Humans are exposed to 89 of these—again, mostly on the job.

How do scientists know that something causes cancer?

Unfortunately, they too often find out by accident when an unexpected number of people who work with a particular substance develop a certain type of cancer. Vinyl chloride is

* **Updated information (July 1977):** A total of 369 chemicals have been evaluated for cancer risk to humans in 16 IARC Monograph volumes. For 25 of these 369 chemicals, definite evidence or strong suspicion of cancer-causing effect was shown in man, while for 171, definite experimental evidence existed.

Industrial Chemicals Believed to Cause (or Suspected of Causing) Cancer in Humans *

Chemical	Target Organ(s)	Route of Exposure
4-Aminobiphenyl	bladder	inhalation, oral
Arsenic compounds	skin, ? lung	oral, inhalation
Asbestos (crocidolite, amosite, chrysolite, and anthophyllite)	lung and chest cavity gastrointestinal tract	inhalation, oral
Auramine	bladder	oral, inhalation, skin
Benzene	bone marrow	inhalation, skin
Benzidine	bladder	inhalation, oral, skin
Bis(chloromethyl)ether	lung	inhalation
Cadmium oxide and sulphate	prostate, ? lung	inhalation, oral
Chromium (chromate-pro-ducing industries)	lung	inhalation
Hematite (mining)	lung	inhalation
2-Naphthylamine	bladder	inhalation, oral
Nickel (nickel refining)	nasal cavity, lung	inhalation
Soot and tars	lung	
Vinyl chloride	skin (scrotum)	skin contact
	liver, brain, lung	inhalation, skin

* This TABLE does not include many other chemicals that have been shown to produce cancers in animals, but whose effects in humans are not definitely known.

an excellent example. As early as 1930, scientists reported that exposure to vinyl chloride caused ill effects in laboratory animals. Over the years numerous studies have found that it can damage the central nervous system, liver, lungs, and bones of the fingers in humans. In 1970, Italian scientists noted that rats exposed to very high levels for one year had developed tumors. But it wasn't until 1974, when a plant physician for B.F. Goodrich announced three cases of a very rare liver cancer among workers at a single vinyl chloride production plant, that vinyl chloride was widely recognized or accepted as a serious cancer hazard.

Workers are too often the guinea pigs. As Dr. J. William Lloyd, formerly with NIOSH and now an epidemiologist with the United Steelworkers, has said, "Almost everything we know now about occupational cancer comes from counting dead bodies."

It doesn't have to be this way. Laboratory tests in which animals are exposed to suspected carcinogens can be relied upon to predict whether those substances are cancer hazards in humans. This is why so many scientists and labor leaders are urging that more testing be done, and why they have so strongly supported the Toxic Substances Control Act, recently passed by Congress. The new law gives the government authority to require that certain chemicals be tested for health hazards *before* they are put on the market.

How do scientists know that something that causes cancer in animals will also cause it in humans?

There are limits to animal tests. For example, reactions may vary among different species, or a chemical that may cause cancer in man might not produce tumors in animals. Nevertheless, animal tests are currently the most reliable tests we have. In fact, arsenic is just about the only substance we know to be carcinogenic in humans that has failed to cause cancer in animals. Often, a carcinogen will cause tumors in the same body organs in both animals and humans. Despite this convincing track record, some persons are still cautious about using results of animal tests to predict effects in man.

There is nothing to suggest that a substance that causes cancer in animals will not, under any circumstances, produce tumors in man. In fact, the reliability of well-done animal tests is considered so good that it has become the basis for government policy. In 1970 a special advisory group reported to the Surgeon General of the United States:

"Any substance which is shown conclusively to cause tumors in animals should be considered carcinogenic and therefore a potential cancer hazard to man."

This principle was the basis for Occupational Safety and Health Administration (OSHA) standards on the chemicals ethyleneamine and 3,3-dichlorobenzidine and Environmental Protection Agency standards on the pesticides aldrin and dieldrin. These regulations, based on animal evidence of a cancer hazard, were upheld by federal courts.

Other official advisory groups have agreed that a substance should be considered carcinogenic even if it causes benign, or noncancerous, tumors in animals, because benign tumors sometimes become malignant. One panel said flatly that it was "unaware of the existence of any chemical which is capable of producing benign tumors only."

The government also has determined, at least where food is concerned, that there is no way of determining a safe level for any substance that has caused cancer in animals. This policy was the basis for the 1958 Delaney clause in the federal Food, Drug and Cosmetic Act, which says that no food additive that has induced cancer in man or animals when eaten can be considered safe at any level.

Unfortunately, there is still no Delaney-type legislation applying to cancer-causing substances in the workplace.

If animal tests are so reliable, why aren't more chemicals being tested?

At present, the law requires only that some drugs and chemicals added to foods be tested for cancer-causing activity. Human beings are exposed to thousands of other natural or man-made chemicals for which the law does not require testing, although the new Toxic Substances Control Act will change that to some degree.

Scientists have listed more than 3 million distinct chemical compounds, but no one knows how many of these chemicals people are exposed to, or how many other unlisted compounds might exist in our environment.

Unfortunately, animal tests for cancer are extremely time-consuming and expensive. Such tests often require that rats or mice be exposed to a substance throughout their lifetimes, which means that it takes roughly two years to test one chemical in just one species. Also, the standard animal tests now cost nearly $200,000 per chemical. It seems unlikely that society will ever allocate enough money and laboratory space for animal testing of all chemicals in the environment. Even if the funds were available, there would probably not be enough trained scientists to accomplish such a task.

The greatest hope for detecting more of the carcinogens in the sea of chemicals around us probably lies in the development of reliable, rapid, short-term, and inexpensive tests. Such tests would be most useful for pinpointing, among the thousands of untested chemicals, those that should receive first priority in the more extensive, long-term animal tests.

The most promising of these new tests is the Ames test, developed by Dr. Bruce Ames of the University of California at Berkeley. In this simple test, bacteria are used to identify whether a chemical is a *mutagen*—that is, whether it causes changes in the genetic material of a cell. The test can be used to identify cancer-causing substances, because almost all carcinogens are also mutagens. So far, about 85 percent of the known carcinogens on which the Ames test has been tried have been detected as mutagens.

Scientists are working on a number of other short-term tests. One test identifies cancer-causing chemicals by how they behave chemically rather than by whether they produce tumors. Another would identify a carcinogen by whether or not it reacts with certain critical molecules within a cell. The reaction of a carcinogen with the DNA, or genetic material, of a cell triggers repair activity to replace the damaged DNA. So, another test under development would focus on this repair mechanism as an indication that a carcinogen had acted on the cell. Yet another test would monitor changes in animal cells that take place in cell cultures after the cells have been exposed to a carcinogen.

None of these tests is yet reliable enough for its results to be depended on absolutely. In the near future, no single test will be the answer to rapid cancer screening. However, scientists think that a combination of short-term tests can be especially useful for identifying substances that should be given quick attention in cancer research. For example, the Ames test has identified most common hair dyes as potent mutagens. Since 20 million people in the United States dye their hair, these chemicals could represent a serious public health hazard if they do indeed cause cancer. The National Cancer Institute and the hair dye industry now are putting these dyes through conventional cancer tests in animals.

Short-term tests could also provide an early warning that a chemical, such as one slated to become a food additive, may be dangerous before it gets very far along the path to going on the market. Or, if an industrial process is being developed that would expose large numbers of workers to a certain chemical unless expensive safety precautions are taken, early indication of a hazard could guide development toward less hazardous alternatives.

We do know that some substances cause cancer in humans or in several kinds of animals. Why aren't these banned?

There have been attempts to do so. Great Britain and Italy, for example, have tried to stop the manufacture of benzidine, an ingredient of dyes that is known to cause bladder cancer in humans, and since OSHA issued a standard on benzidine as part of its standard on 14 carcinogens, its major manufacturers in this country have radically reduced production of this chemical. But a large number of plants that use it in production of dyes are now making their own benzidine, with workers still being exposed. In a sense, the obvious conclusion could be that our society values certain shades of colors for its textiles over the health of its workers—and perhaps over the health of the general population, since benzidine wastes from manufacturing plants were and still may be released into our waterways. At the least, our regulatory agencies and mechanisms have not responded adequately to the urgency of the situation.

The solution, however, cannot be simply the banning of *all* dangerous substances or manufacturing processes (see Chapter 9); economic considerations often must be considered when setting standards or when withdrawing hazardous materials from the market (see Chapter 12). Many labor leaders and scientists argue that if workers were properly informed about cancer hazards, they could press for adequate standards and protective measures in the workplace. Part of the problem is that workers themselves are often the last to know that a particular chemical is hazardous.

Part II
CANCER HAZARDS

The kinds of substances that cause occupational cancer can be divided into three broad categories: chemicals, metals, and dusts and fibers.

They do their damage by acting alone or probably more often by acting in combination with another workplace carcinogen or with cigarette smoke. They can harm people outside as well as inside the factory by clinging to workers' clothes or by seeping into the air of the surrounding neighborhood. As Chapter 7 points out, occupational cancer has a long reach.

The cancer hazards discussed in the next few chapters are by no means the only ones workers have to worry about. They are, however, some of the more common ones that large numbers of workers are exposed to. And they give some idea of the frightening scope of the occupational cancer problem. (To some degree, at least, perhaps the more worrisome ones are those we haven't yet identified—since we then don't know that we should take precautions.)

Chapter 3
Chemicals

In many ways, the workplace is a mystery world. No one really knows what the 20, 30, or 40,000 industrial chemicals introduced as part of manufacturing processes in the past several decades may be doing to workers' health. Scientists know little about which chemicals individually can cause cancer, and they know even less about the hazards posed by combinations of chemicals. Nor do they understand the effects of exposure to a whole string of carcinogens as a worker moves from one job to another, or as manufacturing processes change.

The hope in this grim picture lies in continuing research. The answers are coming too late for many workers, but slowly we *are* learning more about occupational cancer and what causes it. The following sections describe what scientists have discovered recently about some common chemical hazards.

Vinyl chloride

When B.F. Goodrich announced in January 1974 that three workers at its Louisville, Ky., vinyl chloride plant had angiosarcoma, an extremely rare liver cancer, the words "vinyl chloride" almost overnight became synonymous with "occupational cancer."

Even before Goodrich announced this tragedy, other scientists had been finding liver cancer, as well as tumors of the brain, kidney, lung, and lymphatic system, among laboratory animals exposed to vinyl chloride. Unfortunately, this information had not gotten through to workers in the plants. In any case, once the workers' cancers were known, the National Institute for Occupational Safety and Health (NIOSH) decided to study workers at four vinyl chloride plants to get some idea of the extent of the vinyl chloride hazard to humans.

NIOSH selected four plants that had been polymerizing vinyl chloride for between 20 and 32 years. Because of the latent period between exposure to a substance and onset of cancer, the researchers focused their study on people who had worked with vinyl chloride for five years or more and who were first exposed to the chemical at least 10 years ago. NIOSH reviewed employment records and followed up on the 1,294 workers who met these requirements.

The study showed higher-than-expected rates of death from cancer of the brain and central nervous system, respiratory system, liver, and lymph- and blood-forming tissues. The longer the interval since onset of vinyl chloride exposure, the higher the death rates. For example, the rates were higher for those workers who had their first exposure to vinyl chloride 15 years ago than for those who were first exposed 10 years ago. All 11 of the workers at the four plants who had died of angiosarcoma had worked at one time or another as reactor cleaners, jobs that exposed them heavily to vinyl chloride.

The NIOSH researchers concluded that "evidence now points to vinyl chloride" as the cause of the excessive cancer risk found among these workers.

NIOSH also investigated any cancer deaths among former employees of the four plants, regardless of whether the victim had been exposed for five years or had passed the 10-year latency period. In one case, a man who had been exposed to vinyl chloride for only about three years died of angiosarcoma 17 years later at age 41. This is further evidence for the unfortunate fact that cancer is an irreversible process that continues for many years, even after exposure to a carcinogen has ceased.

•   •   •

It is important to note that in some studies of job hazards, including vinyl chloride, scientists have found *fewer* deaths among workers than would be expected in the general population—at least for the first 5–10 years of a study. This is due to what is sometimes called the "healthy worker effect." It means simply that the healthiest members of the population generally are the ones who are employed. People in poor health often choose not to work in certain jobs—especially ones where they must breathe dusts and fumes—or else companies refuse to hire them on the basis of pre-employment medical examinations.

A study of a group of workers can sometimes be overloaded with newly hired employees who would not have started a new job if they had not been in good health. By restricting their vinyl chloride study to workers who were first exposed to vinyl chloride 10 years ago, the NIOSH researchers avoided having their results clouded by the "healthy worker effect."

Anesthetics

The occupational cancer hazard isn't limited just to "Belchfire Industries." It apparently exists even in what should be the cleanest workplace of all—the hospital operating room. There, doctors, anesthesiologists, and nurse anesthetists are regularly exposed to such anesthetic gases as nitrous oxide, halothane, methoxyflurane, trichloroethylene, and enflurane that leak from operating room equipment.

A nationwide survey by NIOSH and the American Society of Anesthesiologists of 50,000 operating room employees shows that these workers, regularly exposed to trace amounts of anesthetics, develop cancer—especially leukemia and lymphoma—1.3 to 2 times as frequently as medical personnel who do not work in operating rooms. A study of 600 nurse anesthetists in Michigan by Dr. Thomas Corbett of the Veterans Administration Hospital in Ann Arbor revealed a cancer rate three times higher than expected.

In both studies, women who worked in operating rooms during pregnancy had higher rates of miscarriages and birth defects among their children than women who were not exposed to anesthetics. In the Michigan study, two children born to nurse anesthetists who had worked during pregnancy developed cancer.

(It is probably more than coincidence that chemists—who, like anesthesiologists, are exposed to low concentrations of volatile chemicals and gases—also have a higher cancer death rate than do other professional groups.)

Several common anesthetics are chemically similar to such known carcinogens as vinyl chloride and bis(chloromethyl) ether, but most of these have never been tested for cancer-causing activity. In one of the few studies that have been done, researchers at the Veterans Administration Hospital in Ann Arbor, Mich., found that young mice developed tumors after exposure to isoflurane, an experimental anesthetic that has not been put on the market. In light of these findings, the researchers say, isoflurane and similar halogenated ether and alkane anesthetics "must now be regarded with suspicion and studied as soon as possible."

Bis(chloromethyl)ether

Bis(chloromethyl)ether (BCME, also called dichlorodimethyl ether), an alkylating agent used in a variety of industrial synthesis processes, and also used to kill bacteria and fungi, ranks high among potent carcinogens in the workplace.

On the basis of a lung cancer survey and sputum cytology tests at an anion-exchange resin plant in California, NIOSH concluded that workers exposed to BCME have an unusually high risk of cancer.

The sputum cytology test, in which coughed-up samples of sputum are analyzed under the microscope, can sometimes detect lung damage and even lung cancer before it shows up on an x-ray. In the California study, 34 percent of the workers who had been exposed to BCME for five years or more had abnormal lung cells in their sputum. Only 11 percent of those in a control group not exposed to BCME had abnormal cells.

NIOSH also found that the 136 employees who had been exposed to BCME for five years or more had nine times the normal risk of lung cancer. The reported cases of lung cancer occurred among relatively young men—average age 47—who had had an average of 10 years' exposure to BCME.

Most of the lung cancer victims smoked cigarettes, which indicates that cigarette smoke may have "promoted" the effect of the carcinogen, as is the case for asbestos workers and uranium miners. The evidence, however, points to BCME, not cigarette smoke, as the chief cause of the lung cancers, because the disease struck nonsmokers as well as smokers. It also occurred at a younger age and was a different type of lung cancer from that usually caused by smoking.

NIOSH's findings of a high lung cancer risk among BCME workers are supported by other studies, such as one which showed that workers exposed to BCME in a Philadelphia chemical plant had eight times the rate of lung cancer as people not exposed to the substance. Researchers from the Institute of Environmental Medicine at New York University recently studied 1,800 workers exposed for at least five years to chloromethyl methyl ether (CMME), which is usually contaminated with two-to-eight percent BCME. These workers died from lung cancer at a rate two-and-a-half times that of a control group.

•   •   •

Knowledge of the BCME hazard grew dramatically when scientists reported recently that the vapors of hydrochloric acid and formaldehyde—two chemicals found together in many industrial situations—can combine spontaneously to form BCME.

In a survey of various workplaces, NIOSH found that small concentrations of BCME were forming in the textile industry. NIOSH now is working with the industry to eliminate the possibility of further contamination. The Institute also is checking whether BCME is forming in such other places as biological and chemical laboratories, insect-rearing laboratories, and particleboard and paper manufacturing plants, where hydrochloric acid and formaldehyde are commonly found together.

In light of the BCME discovery, NIOSH experts warn that these two chemicals should not be used in the same place except under very well-controlled conditions.

Coke-oven emissions and coke by-products

An extensive study of 58,800 men employed at seven Pittsburgh area steel plants showed that working on or near coke ovens is one of the most dangerous jobs around. The most startling discovery was that full-time topside oven workers with five or more years' exposure are almost 11 times as likely to get lung cancer as are other steel workers. For side-oven workers, the risk is two-and-a-half times as great.

This study, by the University of Pittsburgh School of Public Health and NIOSH, found that *all* coke-plant workers—not just those on the ovens—have higher rates of cancer than do other steel workers. Non-oven workers have less chance of getting lung cancer but fall prey to cancers of the digestive system, especially of the colon and pancreas. Cancers of the mouth and throat also are common.

Although the primary purpose of a coke plant is to transform coal into coke for use in blast furnaces, a secondary function is to recover chemical by-products that result from the carbonization of bituminous coal. Various aromatic amines present in the by-products area of a coke plant—such as benzpyrene, anthracene, benzol, coal tar and pitch, and creosote—are known to cause cancer. Some aromatic amines found in the coke plant specifically cause colon cancer in laboratory rats.

Although coke-oven emissions have attracted the most attention because of disastrously high cancer rates among coke-oven workers, cancer hazards in the rest of the coke plant cannot be ignored.

Benzene

For more than a century, scientists have known that benzene is a powerful bone marrow poison, causing such conditions as aplastic anemia. In the past several decades, evidence has been mounting that benzene may also cause leukemia.

The first case of "benzene leukemia" was identified in 1928 in a worker so heavily exposed to the solvent that his fellow workers could stand no more than two months in the same job without becoming ill. Worldwide, there are now *at least* 150 documented cases of leukemia attributed to exposure to benzene.

Italian scientists report that many cases of leukemia have shown up among workers in rotogravure and shoe manufacturing plants where there had been outbreaks of benzene poisoning before Italy banned the use of benzene in 1963. The risk of leukemia among former workers in these factories is at least 20 times higher than for the general population.

These scientists note that aplastic anemia usually occurs while workers are still exposed to high concentrations of benzene. But leukemia may not show up until many years later.

One woman who suffered from typical benzene anemia in 1957 had almost normal blood counts for 14 years. Then in 1972 she was stricken with leukemia and died five months later. Despite the lag in the development of leukemia, her disease is still considered occupational cancer.

Since the Italian rotogravure industry began using toluene as a solvent instead of benzene, no cases of job-related leukemia or aplastic anemia have turned up.

Another interesting study of benzene and leukemia comes from Japan. A survey of leukemia cases among adult survivors of the atomic bomb blasts at Hiroshima and Nagasaki showed that the risk of leukemia was two-and-a-half times higher among those bomb survivors who had a history of job exposure to benzene or medical x-rays.

In the United States, a major source of exposure to benzene has been in the rubber industry, where benzene was once the most commonly used solvent. A recent study by the University of North Carolina School of Public Health of causes of death among workers in various jobs within the rubber industry showed that those who were exposed to solvents have three times the normal risk of leukemia. Those exposed to high levels of solvents have a risk five times higher than normal.

Other chemicals in the rubber industry

The rubber tire manufacturing industry uses a vast and ever-changing variety of chemicals. Besides benzene, the known or suspected carcinogens now in use or used in the past include beta-naphthylamine, talc dust containing asbestos, and various nitrosamines. When certain substances are subjected to very high temperatures, as is required in several rubber manufacturing processes, any number of unidentified chemicals are released.

The hazards of working in the rubber industry have been recognized for decades. The British reported in the early 1930s that rubber workers had a higher-than-average cancer death rate. In 1950 the U.S. government found that rubber workers had a rate of cancer deaths eight percent higher than that of workers in other manufacturing industries. The most common cancers were those of the large bowel, respiratory system, and lymph- and blood-forming tissues. A recently completed study, however, has shed more light than ever on the causes of cancer in the rubber industry.

Through an occupational health research program negotiated in 1970 by the United Rubber Workers and four major rubber companies—Firestone, Goodyear, General Tire and Rubber, and Uniroyal—scientists from the University of North Carolina School of Public Health have been studying causes of death among rubber workers during the past 10 years. They have attempted to link certain types of cancer with specific jobs and, where possible, with specific chemicals. Their study has revealed a higher-than-expected number of deaths from cancer in general and especially high rates of cancer of the stomach, colon, prostate, and lymph- and blood-forming systems.

Besides linking leukemia to solvent exposure, the study has indicated a connection between lung cancer and working in the curing room. Stomach cancer was most common among people who had worked in compounding, mixing and milling, and in jobs involving contact with "green rubber." Scientists now are conducting a detailed study of possible causes of stomach cancer, which they think might be the result of swallowing carbon black—a compound containing such carcinogens as benzpyrene —as well as asbestos and nitrosamines.

Bladder cancer is most prevalent among workers at the beginning of the production line, in jobs such as shipping and receiving, compounding, mixing, milling, and calendering.

These are jobs in which workers are most likely to come into contact with raw-ingredient chemicals.

There is no clear association between specific jobs and prostate cancer. However, such cancers did occur among workers in the compounding and mixing areas, where metallic oxides are used as accelerators in the vulcanizing process. Among these is cadmium oxide. In the past, cadmium has been linked to prostate cancer (see Chapter 4).

Chloroprene

Chloroprene is an example of a potential cancer hazard that was discovered as a direct result of the vinyl chloride tragedy. Introduced by Du Pont in 1931, it is used mainly in the manufacture of a synthetic rubber known as neoprene. For years, scientists have known that chloroprene can act as a depressant on the central nervous system and can harm the lungs, liver, and kidneys. But it had never been associated with cancer.

When the news broke about vinyl chloride, industry and government scientists began to take a closer look at workers exposed to chemicals—such as chloroprene—that are very similar in chemical structure to vinyl chloride and that are also known to cause liver damage.

Du Pont reviewed the health records and death certificates of its employees who had worked with chloroprene and found that the number of lung cancers had increased in recent years. After further analysis, however, the company concluded that the increase was not connected with job exposures.

Fortunately, Du Pont's cancer research efforts include keeping track of studies from other countries. A survey of foreign scientific literature turned up two reports from the Soviet Union that linked exposure to chloroprene with unusually high rates of lung and skin cancer. The incidence of cancer increased dramatically with the length of time a worker was exposed, the Soviets found.

In light of these findings, Du Pont and NIOSH have launched a detailed study of causes of death among all people who ever worked with chloroprene. Du Pont has also started long-term studies to determine if chloroprene causes cancer in animals.

Benzpyrene

Benzpyrene (benzo[a]pyrene), or BaP for short, is an ingredient of cigarette smoke and city air that is known to cause cancer in animals. This suggested the possibility that BaP in cigarette smoke might account for the high degree of association between cigarette smoking and lung cancer as well as contribute to higher lung cancer rates among city dwellers.

Roofers and waterproofers, who work with hot pitch and asphalt, are exposed to far greater amounts of BaP than even heavy cigarette smokers who live in urban areas. To find out about the effects of heavy doses of BaP on these workers, scientists from the American Cancer Society and the Mount Sinai School of Medicine in New York traced nearly 6,000 members of the United Slate, Tile and Composition Roofers, Damp and Waterproof Workers' Association, which has locals in all parts of the United States.

They found that roofers and waterproofers regularly exposed to BaP, especially those who have been working with pitch and asphalt for 20 years or more, have significantly higher death rates from lung cancer, as well as from cancers of the mouth and lip, throat, larynx, and esophagus.

The scientists say it is difficult to pin the blame solely on BaP, since fumes from hot pitch contain a number of substances. Also, many of the roofers smoked, and it is possible that the very high rate of lung cancer after 20 years on the job was partly the result of BaP and cigarette smoke acting together. Nevertheless, the evidence is convincing enough that BaP retains its reputation as an occupational cancer hazard.

Cutting and lubricating oils

There is a great deal of evidence that various types of mineral oil cause skin cancer. In the 1920s, scientists reported so-called paraffin cancers among Scottish and European workers involved in the refining of shale oil, coal oil, and petroleum. Men working as "mule spinners" in the British cotton textile industry have a high rate of scrotal cancer, apparently from continuous bodily contact with oils used to lubricate machinery. Machine operators exposed to lubricating and cooling fluids while cutting and grinding metals have gotten cancers of the hands, arms, and scrotum.

Since the violent action of moving parts during machining operations releases oil mists and vapors into the air, scientists have long been concerned that inhaling these mists could pose an additional cancer hazard for workers. One NIOSH study of some 5,200 people who worked in metal machining jobs for at least one year revealed no unusually high death rates from cancer of the lungs or digestive system.

A very recent report from NIOSH, however, raises a new red flag about industrial oils. Scientists have found that oils used by an estimated 780,000 industrial workers to reduce heat and friction during metal machining operations contain significant amounts of nitrosamines, known cancer-causing substances. Most cutting oils, now largely synthetic, contain both nitrites and amines that are added for such purposes as inhibiting rust. Studies indicate that these two substances combine in the oils to form "relatively massive amounts" of nitrosamines.

Chapter 4
Metals

Mining and smelting of metals was one of the earliest industrial activities known to man. The ability to process metals has been a keystone in the development of civilization. But even the ancient Romans noted that in terms of workers' health, the costs were staggering.

The dangers of metals, especially lead, have been known for more than one thousand years. But with the exception of arsenic, the association between metals and cancer dates back only about 50 years. Since then, many metals or metallic compounds have been shown to cause cancer in animals. These include beryllium, cadmium, chromium, cobalt, iron, lead, nickel, selenium, zinc, and titanium. Some metals—notably nickel, arsenic, and chromates—are potent carcinogens in man.

Metals are of special concern because they occur naturally in the environment. Therefore, a worker's exposure does not end with the eight-hour workday. He/she continues to be exposed to metals in the air, food, and water. Since the body is slow in removing many metals, they may accumulate in tissues and produce long-range effects.

Another reason for concern is the ability of such metals as lead and mercury to cross the placenta of a pregnant woman and harm her unborn child. This particular hazard has led some experts to suggest that women capable of bearing children be barred from jobs where lead, for example, is used. The solution, of course, is not to restrict certain jobs just to the hardiest individuals in the population. Rather, employers have a responsibility under the law to clean up the workplace and make it safe for *all* workers.

In any consideration of the link between metals and cancer, it is important to note that metal workers are exposed not only to various metals and metallic compounds but also to silica, lubricants, chemical fumes, and other agents that might cause cancer. Nevertheless, the high rates of cancer among workers throughout the metals industry point to the hazards of metals themselves.

In Japan, for example, the number of lung cancer deaths among metal workers far exceeds the number expected for the average population. Stomach cancer also is prevalent. As the following sections describe, various groups of workers in the American metals industry also are dying from cancer far more frequently than expected.

A survey of 10 occupational groups

Dr. Samuel Milham of the Washington State Department of Social and Health Services has studied, by statistical means, cancer deaths among 10 groups of metal workers in the State of Washington—boilermakers, copper smelter workers, machinists, metal molders, plumbers, structural metal workers, sheet metal workers, aluminum mill workers, welders, and tool-and-die makers—and has found that all 10 have high rates of respiratory cancer. This is in line with evidence that such metals as nickel, arsenic, and chromates cause lung cancer in humans.

Four groups—boilermakers, plumbers, structural metal workers, and welders—also appear to be susceptible to bladder cancer. Cancer of the tongue is evident among machinists, plumbers, and structural metal workers. Aluminum mill workers and sheet metal workers have high rates of pancreatic cancer. Malignant lymphoma was common among aluminum mill workers and plumbers.

The cancers among aluminum mill workers seem to be concentrated among potroom employees, who are exposed to coal tar pitch volatiles. Researchers suspect that these substances, rather than metals, may be most responsible for the cancers among this group of workers.

Cancer in the steel industry

Some studies of the steel industry indicate that cancer hazards are pretty well limited to coke plants and particularly to the coke-oven areas. However, a study by Dr. Edward Radford of Johns Hopkins University of workers in a large Baltimore steel plant, which revealed high rates of bladder, respiratory, and kidney cancer, has shed new light on hazards in the steel industry. Most surprising was the discovery of numerous lung cancer cases among workers in steel-finishing operations.

These findings suggest that cancer-causing agents may be more widespread in steel manufacturing than had previously been thought, although the study does not link the cancers with specific substances. Scientists point out that the steel industry, like most industries, is constantly introducing new processes, which can mean worker exposure to countless new substances. Changes are perhaps most frequent in steel-finishing operations.

This highlights an important point about occupational cancer: the fact that past studies showed no increased cancer risk does not necessarily mean that trouble will not show up later in the same industry. Cancer hazards change along with technological change.

Arsenic

Forty-five years after Percivall Pott discovered scrotal cancer among chimney sweeps, another English physician, J. A. Paris, reported seeing "a cancerous disease in the scrotum, similar to that which infests chimney sweeps" among men exposed to arsenic fumes in a copper smelter. The doctor's observation was never confirmed, however, and is still the subject of dispute and controversy.

But by 1930, scientists knew definitely that workers manufacturing sheep dip, a veterinary pesticide containing arsenic, were prone to skin cancer. In 1934, doctors judged that inhaling arsenic might be responsible for lung cancer among sheep-dip workers. Later studies revealed high rates of lung

cancer among metal industry workers involved in copper smelting and production of arsenic trioxide and lymphatic cancer
among workers manufacturing arsenic pesticides.

In one National Cancer Institute study of copper smelter
workers, lung cancer deaths increased steadily with the length
of exposure to arsenic, ranging from two to five times the
expected rate. The greatest number of lung cancer deaths
occurred among those workers exposed both to arsenic and
sulfur dioxide, which suggests that sulfur dioxide may be a
co-carcinogen that enhances the cancer-causing effects of arsenic.

Cadmium

Some 100,000 workers in the United States are exposed to
cadmium, which is used in the electroplating industry, the
rubber industry, in nickel-cadmium batteries, brazing-soldering
alloys, pigments and chemicals, and as a stabilizer in plastics.
A number of studies in the past have indicated that cadmium
causes cancer in both humans and animals.

This conclusion was supported by a recent NIOSH survey
of nearly 300 men who had worked at least two years in a
cadmium smelter. These workers had significantly higher death
rates from all forms of cancer, especially cancers of the lung
and prostate gland. Lung cancer occurred at more than twice
the expected rate, and as with many other occupational cancers, the risk of developing the disease increased with the
length of time after exposure to the metal began. Workers first
exposed to cadmium 20 or more years ago ran an especially
significant risk of prostate cancer.

Lead

One of the best known and most studied of occupational
hazards, lead has been recognized as a poison for about one
thousand years. Although some recent studies link lead with
cancer, this metal apparently is not a potent carcinogen in
humans.

In one study by Tabershaw/Cooper Associates, Inc. of
Berkeley, California, over 7,000 men who had worked for at

least one year in a lead smelter or lead battery plant and who had been heavily exposed to the metal had only slightly higher than expected rates of cancer of the lung, stomach, and large intestine. Although in other studies, animals fed large amounts of lead salts developed kidney tumors, this survey of smelter and battery plant workers turned up no unusually high numbers of urinary tract cancers.

Of concern, however, is a practice in the lead industry of giving workers drugs known as chelating agents in order to reduce the levels of lead in their blood. This often gives the impression that they are exposed to much lower levels of lead then they actually are.

Chapter 5
Dusts and Fibers

"Dust" is a catch-all category, because cancer hazards associated with dusts can involve many different kinds of substances. Dusts that workers breathe may carry materials—such as radioactive particles or asbestos fibers—that are the actual cause of cancer. In some situations—the high incidence of cancer among woodworkers, for example—scientists don't know whether the dust itself is responsible for the disease or whether chemicals or breakdown products common in the industry are the culprits.

But whether the dust or the substances carried by the dust are to blame, there is evidence that dusts present in a number of industries contribute significantly to occupational cancer. The following are several examples of dangerous dusts.

Asbestos

One of the best known occupational hazards is asbestos, a fibrous mineral that has been widely used for insulation and fireproofing, in textiles, and in cement and drywall compounds.

The suggestion that asbestos could cause cancer was first raised in 1935 by two doctors, K. M. Lynch and W. A. Smith, who had noticed an association between asbestosis, an often fatal fibrosis of the lung, and lung cancer. The link between asbestos exposure and lung cancer was established definitely around 1955.

By 1960, asbestos was recognized as the cause of mesothelioma, a rare and always fatal cancer of the membranes that surround the lungs and line the abdominal cavity. Higher-than-normal rates of gastrointestinal cancer also have been found among American insulation workers. And, most recently, asbestos has been linked with cancer of the larynx. Today, we have evidence to show that cigarette smokers with heavy asbestos exposure may be 90 times more likely than the average nonsmoker to develop lung cancer.

Even relatively brief exposures can increase the risk of cancer 20, 30, or 40 years later. Dr. Irving Selikoff of Mount Sinai School of Medicine explains:

"A worker could be exposed heavily to asbestos for even one day and conceivably develop cancer much later in life as a result of this exposure. He may have been exposed for only one day, but his lungs continue to be exposed to the asbestos deposited there."

Consequently, scientists estimate that of the 1 million current and former asbestos workers in the United States, 300,000 to 400,000 can be expected to die of cancer—one in five from lung cancer, one in 10 from cancer of the gastrointestinal tract, and one in 20 from mesothelioma.

All commercial forms of asbestos have been linked with cancer, and recent studies among hard-rock gold miners indicate that noncommercial forms—present as contaminants in other products, such as commercial talc, as well as in the air in many parts of the United States—also are capable of causing cancer.

The same studies showed that fibers shorter than five micrometers ($\frac{1}{200}$th of a millimeter) in length can also cause cancer and nonmalignant respiratory disease. Until now, most concern has centered on fibers longer than five micrometers.

Fibrous glass

In recent years, fibrous glass has replaced asbestos in many insulation and fireproofing materials. Since fibrous glass, like asbestos, is made up of tiny fibers, scientists naturally are concerned about whether inhaling it can cause cancer. Studies in the past have produced conflicting results, in part because, unlike natural fibers, the physical characteristics of glass fiber can and do change continuously according to use.

Since commercial production and use of fibrous glass in the United States date back only to about 1933, it wasn't until recently that sufficient time had lapsed for job-related cancers to start showing up. Since various studies had shown that fibrous glass causes cancer in experimental animals and that a large number of fibrous glass workers were retiring on disability because of chronic bronchitis, NIOSH launched a major study of disease and death in the fibrous glass manufacturing industry.

NIOSH's survey of causes of death among 1,448 workers exposed to low levels of airborne glass fibers revealed a high rate of nonmalignant respiratory disease. There was *no* excess risk of lung cancer among these workers, even 20 years after first exposure.

Another part of the study, however, did indicate some increased risk of cancer among workers involved during the early years of fibrous glass production with a special process that created exposure to glass particles of very small diameter. Since small-diameter fibers also have caused cancer in animals, scientists still are reserving judgment on the safety of fibrous glass, especially since most fibrous glass manufactured in the *past* was thick—too thick to enter the recesses of the lung. Now, thinner fibers are being produced, and scientists stress that until more is known, exposure to glass fibers should be kept to a minimum through engineering controls and good work practices.

Radioactive dusts

Radiation is a unique cancer hazard. Since it is a form of energy rather than, say, a chemical or metal, it really doesn't fit into any of our hazard categories. Radioactive particles, however, can be borne by dust, creating a serious hazard for workers who breathe the dust. This hazard particularly affects underground miners.

A lung disease "epidemic" among mine workers was first mentioned in 1556 by Georgius Agricola, a municipal physician for a mining village in Central Europe. Agricola observed that the "miners' disease" affected miners after about 10 years of working underground and that it was responsible for 30 to 70 percent of miners' deaths in that area. Three centuries after Agricola, 75 percent of the deaths among miners in his small village still were caused by the same disease: lung cancer.

At first, arsenic in the ore was thought to be the cause of the miners' cancer. But scientists now recognize that an even more potent carcinogen—radon—was responsible. This radioactive gas is produced by the natural decay of uranium and radium, but its presence is by no means limited to uranium and radium deposits. It can exist in a variety of metal and non-metal mines. The Mining Enforcement and Safety Administration reports that in the United States, measurable amounts of radon have been found in mines producing clay, iron, fluorspar, tungsten, copper, and zinc.

Radon escapes from rock into open areas of a mine. When a miner inhales it, his whole body is in effect exposed to radiation. The hazard is limited, though, because most radon is exhaled within its half-life of 3.8 days. Far more dangerous are the radon "daughters," or decay products of radon. These radionuclides, which have an average half-life of 30 minutes, quickly attach to solid surfaces—like dust particles. When miners inhale these dust particles, the radiation attacks those areas in the nose, throat, and lungs where the dust particles are deposited. The dose of radiation a uranium miner's lungs receive from these dust particles is 20 times greater than from inhaled radon.

Studies have clearly shown that the risk of lung cancer among American uranium miners is directly related to the extent of their exposure to radon "daughters." Until recently there was some question about whether the same lung cancer risk also exists for nonwhite miners—mostly American Indians —and for miners who do not smoke.

A NIOSH follow-up study of causes of death among both

white and Indian miners showed that the lung cancer rate among both races was more than four times the expected rate. The risk was high also for miners who did not smoke or who smoked only a little, although it was not nearly as high as for the heavy smokers.

Wood dust

Under NIOSH contract, a study of nearly 300,000 death records in the State of Washington by Dr. Samuel Milham of the Washington State Department of Social and Health Services has revealed that workers in the wood products industry have unusually high rates of certain types of cancer. Although types of cancer varied among specific occupations, nearly all the groups surveyed—carpenters, loggers, professional foresters, pulp and paper mill workers, and plywood mill workers—had high rates of cancer of the stomach and of the lymph- and blood-forming tissues.

Milham thinks the stomach cancer could result from swallowing wood particles. The blood-and lymphatic-system cancers, especially among pulp and paper mill workers and plywood mill workers, might be caused by chemical breakdown products of wood.

Other types of cancer that showed up among the various occupational groups included: loggers—prostate cancer; professional foresters (who have a variety of exposures in mills and offices, as well as forests)—cancers of the rectum, pancreas, and lungs; pulp and paper mill workers—cancer of the small intestine; and workers in sawmills and other wood-machining operations—cancers of the pancreas and testes. One interesting finding is that people who work in sawmills or where wood is simply machined do not have as high a cancer risk as those in the paper, pulp, and plywood industries.

Obviously, all these groups have one thing in common: they work with wood. Do these results, then, mean that wood causes cancer? There is some fairly convincing evidence from other studies. The British, for example, have found cancer of the nasal passages and sinuses among furniture workers. No such cancers turned up in the Washington study, but British workers handle mostly hardwoods, while the Washington workers dealt mainly with softwoods. Another recent study has indicated that cedar can cause cancer in laboratory mice.

Swedish scientists have discovered an extraordinarily high rate of sinus cancer among woodworkers in that country and numerous stomach cancers among those woodworkers who live in urban areas. Approximately 45 percent of the nasal sinus cancers recorded in the Swedish cancer registry occurred among woodworkers.

Whatever the actual carcinogen—wood dust itself, a breakdown product of wood, or some chemical used in processing or treating wood—the evidence clearly points to a high cancer risk for workers throughout the wood products industry.

Dusts in the textile industry

Textile manufacturing is a dusty business, and by far the dustiest part of the process is the cleaning of the raw fibers. Raw wool, for instance, may contain up to 55 percent non-fibrous material. This "dirt" is removed from the raw wool and raw cotton by beating and crushing it into fine particles that are shaken out and blown or sucked away. Naturally, a good deal of that dust finds its way into workers' noses, mouths, and throats. It isn't too surprising, then, that cancers of the tongue, mouth, and throat were found to be common among textile workers, in one British study.

This study showed that deaths from these cancers were far more common among male textile workers than among men in the general population in England and Wales. Among fiber preparers, the rate was three times higher than for the general population. And the risk appears to be much higher for those who worked with wool than with cotton. (Raw wool often contains residues of sheep dip, a pesticide containing arsenic.)

The Department of Occupational Health at the University of Manchester is conducting a detailed study of disease among workers in the two main textile regions of England—one producing mainly cotton, the other mainly wool. So far, the study has shown that oral and throat cancers found among male textile workers also are common among women employed in the cotton industry. Scientists say the cancers cannot be blamed on such things as wearing dentures, smoking, drinking, or chewing regularly on bits of cotton.

Chapter 6
The Effects of Smoking

It's hardly a secret that smoking is hazardous to your health. Every pack of cigarettes and every cigarette ad contains just such a warning. Many scientists believe smoking is largely responsible for the high rate of lung cancer in this country. And there is little doubt that it increases the cancer risk disproportionately for workers exposed to other carcinogens on the job. Some industries would like to blame most occupational cancer on smoking, but obviously the situation isn't that simple.

Just what is the effect of smoking? It plays a very definite role in certain occupational cancers. As pointed out in earlier chapters on specific cancer hazards, cancer rates among workers exposed to certain workplace carcinogens usually are higher for those who smoke. This is certainly true for uranium miners and for workers exposed to such chemicals as bis(chloromethyl)ether and benzpyrene. Scientists believe that cigarette smoke acts as a co-carcinogen, promoting the cancer-causing effects of some chemicals and dusts.

Among asbestos workers, those who smoke are far more likely (eight times) to get lung cancer and cancer of the esophagus. The combination of asbestos exposure and smoking greatly multiplies the risk of lung cancer.

As far as most occupational health experts are concerned, the message for workers is clear: DON'T SMOKE. Especially those people who work with substances that may already increase their chances of getting cancer should not smoke.

Does this mean that certain "high-risk" industries should not hire people who smoke? Such a drastic policy has been seriously proposed. But that's hardly the answer. Smoking certainly plays a role in development of cancers of the lung, larynx, esophagus, mouth, and throat among some workers. In other occupational cancers, it plays a very minor role.

There seems to be no link, for example, between smoking and the always fatal mesothelioma among asbestos workers. Nor is there any connection between smoking and the risk of colon, rectal, or stomach cancer. The fact that lung cancer occurs among nonsmokers exposed to job hazards, and that it strikes at a younger age than is usually the case just from smoking, indicates that cigarette smoke is not the chief culprit in occupational cancer, but it adds to a bad situation.

Even if you have smoked for years, you can at least decrease your cancer risk by stopping immediately. But banning every cigarette in the country isn't going to eliminate occupational cancer. Only cleaning up the workplace will accomplish that.

Chapter 7
Beyond the Factory Gates

Job health hazards respect no boundaries. There is disturbing evidence that the industrial cancer risk can reach well beyond the factory, endangering workers' families and other residents of the community. Specific studies show that asbestos, vinyl chloride, beryllium, and arsenic already are associated with death and disease among people who never worked with these substances.

Asbestos

Scientists from nine countries have reported a total of nearly 40 cases of mesothelioma—the rare cancer of the membranes lining the lungs and abdominal cavity—among people whose only known exposure to asbestos was living in the home of an asbestos worker. Others have occurred among people who lived near an asbestos factory.

To study the extent of this family risk, investigators from New York City's Mount Sinai School of Medicine examined 326 relatives of asbestos workers from one plant who had their first household contact with asbestos 25 or 30 years ago.

X-rays revealed evidence of asbestos-related disease of the lungs in 35 percent of the relatives. Four cases of mesothelioma have shown up, and two of the victims already have died.*

* By 1977, all had died.

Since many of the people in the study are under age 50, they have many more high-risk years ahead.

The mesothelioma victims included:

- The 40-year-old son of a man who had worked in the asbestos plant for three years until the son was 11 years old.
- The daughter of the plant's chief engineer, 41 years old when she died.
- The 42-year-old daughter of a man who had worked in the plant for five years. When she was 10, she took lunch to her father at the plant every day.
- A 32-year-old woman who at age 13 lived in the home of her brother-in-law while he worked at the plant for six months. Before that, she lived near the plant and often played in the homes of friends whose fathers worked there.

"I really regard these deaths as occupational deaths," comments Dr. Muriel Newhouse of the London School of Hygiene and Tropical Medicine. "If the factory weren't there, they wouldn't have been exposed to asbestos."

Asbestos is particularly hazardous because, once in the house, it is difficult to remove. The dust has been found in homes of some former asbestos workers 20 years after the plant where they worked had closed.

Scientists stress that under no circumstances should asbestos workers bring their dusty clothes home, even to be laundered. The plant should provide adequate changing and showering facilities for workers, and work clothes should be washed by a commercial industrial laundry equipped to handle contaminated clothing. But even this is not an adequate solution *because mesothelioma has also occurred among laundry workers handling the clothes*. A better solution would be to control the dust at *the source*.

Vinyl chloride

Some studies have suggested that wives of vinyl chloride workers have higher than normal rates of miscarriages and stillbirths, but this has been hard to prove because there have been no satisfactory nationwide statistics on miscarriages.

Ohio, however, has required since 1968 that information

about specific birth defects be included on birth certificates. Because of these records, the Industrial Union Department of the AFL-CIO requested Dr. Peter Infante of the Ohio Department of Health to use this information to investigate birth defects in three Ohio cities—Painesville, Ashtabula, and Avon Lake—where vinyl chloride production plants are located.

The study showed that for the entire state, a birth defect occurred in 10.14 of every 1,000 live births. In the three cities having vinyl chloride facilities, however, the rate ranged from 17.37 to 20.33 per 1,000 live births. When data for all three cities were combined, the rate of birth defects was much higher than expected. The rates in these three cities also were way above those in the remainder of the counties where the cities are located.

Dr. Infante found an especially high incidence of defects of the central nervous system, upper digestive tract, and genital organs. Clubfoot also was common. Because of their severity, the central nervous system defects were of most concern.

Interestingly, an analysis of death certificates revealed a large number of deaths from central nervous system tumors among adult men—especially in the same communities that had the highest rate of birth defects of the central nervous system.

Dr. Infante cautioned that these findings don't point definitely to vinyl chloride as the cause of increased birth defects and adult cancers in the three cities. However, he could find no evidence that such factors as the mother's age or race or variations in hospital recordkeeping accounted for the high rates of birth defects. And he noted that the connection between birth defects and adult cancers affecting the same body system should be explored further.

Arsenic

High rates of lung cancer have been found among both men and women in two Montana cities with copper mining and smelting facilities. The best explanation seems to be that the same agent, probably airborne arsenic, which the men are exposed to on the job, has also polluted the community air, contributing to a rise in lung cancer among the women.

Part III
PREVENTING
OCCUPATIONAL CANCER

Setting standards and exposure levels enforceable by law, substituting less dangerous chemicals for known carcinogens, keeping close watch on those workers known to be at high risk of cancer—these are a few approaches to preventing, or at least controlling, the occupational cancer epidemic in this country.

Given the grim statistics and long lists of hazards cited earlier in this book, we obviously have a long way to go. But the following chapters give some indication of what is being done to protect workers from cancer hazards on the job.

Chapter 8
What the Government Is Doing

Scientific understanding of occupational cancer has been growing at a snail's pace compared to what is needed. And the ability of our national organizations—both government and nongovernment—to deal with cancer control has been even slower to develop. As a nation, we still react to crisis situations such as occurred with vinyl chloride instead of preventing them. And we're not even reacting fast enough.

The United States, which is usually considered the most technically advanced nation, might appear to lag behind other countries in protecting workers. Some countries have banned known carcinogens; we are still attempting to set a "safe" level for them. The U.S. Congress, after years of haggling, only recently passed a Toxic Substances Control Act to give the federal government some authority over what chemicals go on the market.

In its efforts to control occupational cancer, the federal government has been handicapped in several ways:

- By the lack of a national consensus to fund research to eliminate or control cancer.

- By the multiplicity of individual agencies with separate authorities and separate approaches to cancer control.

- By major gaps in data available to the government and in the government's power to require data from private industry. (The Toxic Substances Control Act should go a long way toward closing these gaps.)

50

- By the long latent period for occupational cancer, which makes causes and effects difficult to identify and prove. This problem is compounded by the fact that our laws are oriented toward dealing with immediate health effects. The general public, also crisis-oriented, has only recently started to appreciate the dangers of diseases such as cancer that require long periods to develop.

Regulation and research

Ultimately, the job of the federal government is to control cancer hazards through the force of law. The process of regulating dangerous substances has four basic steps: First, the government must gather information about the hazard. Doctors, chemists, statisticians, and others collect data and estimate who is being exposed to what levels of the carcinogen in question. Economists determine how much it will cost to control these exposures and how much will be saved if controls are imposed. Engineers determine possible control technology including product substitution and/or redesigned manufacturing processes. Economic considerations are usually built into the engineering designs.

At the second stage, the government regulators enter to make decisions about control, presumably with full consideration of the public interest. Step three is the actual control, making a standard that exists on paper a reality in the workplace. The fourth step is follow-up, assuring that the standard is being implemented and that the public is getting its money's worth from the regulatory agency charged with controlling the hazard. Too often this last step is neglected or misunderstood. Regulatory efforts are often criticized for being inflationary, but true cost and benefit analyses have never been successfully done (see Chapter 12).

The most visible of the federal agencies involved in controlling occupational cancer are the two created by the 1970 Occupational Safety and Health Act: the Occupational Safety and Health Administration (OSHA) within the Department of Labor, which sets and enforces health and safety standards in the nation's workplaces; and the National Institute for Occupational Safety and Health (NIOSH), an agency of the Department of Health, Education, and Welfare that conducts research on job hazards and recommends new standards to OSHA.

Protecting mine and mill workers is the concern of the Mining Enforcement and Safety Administration (MESA), an agency of the Department of the Interior created in 1973 as the OSHA of the mineral industry. Like OSHA, MESA sets standards and enforces them through inspections.

Also extremely important in federal cancer control is the National Cancer Institute (NCI), part of the National Institutes of Health. Although it is strictly a research agency and not involved in regulation, the results of its scientific research should guide NIOSH and OSHA in making decisions that can become law. As far back as 1948, NCI established an Environmental Cancer Section, headed by Dr. Wilhelm C. Hueper, one of the foremost experts in occupational cancer.

The National Institutes of Health have a number of activities in the area of job-related cancer. These include studies of cancer deaths among selected high-risk groups of workers; assembling information on production, use, and worker exposure to industrial chemicals; long-term animal tests to determine which substances cause cancer; and test-tube studies to find out how living cells respond to a substance—research that it is hoped will lead to rapid cancer screening methods for widely used chemicals.

In the past, carcinogens often were identified only after high cancer rates were seen among people who had been exposed to them. The human danger was then confirmed by animal tests. In the past few years, a new trend has begun to appear: when animal tests have indicated that a chemical causes cancer, the laboratory results are then confirmed by studies of death and disease among exposed workers.

Tragically, it is too late for many victims, but scientists now feel confident that cancer in laboratory animals is a serious warning signal that a substance also will cause cancer in humans. Once a chemical is identified as a carcinogen in animals, it should become a high priority to find out how many people and which people—either on the job or in the community—are exposed to it.

A NIOSH policy on cancer

It is NIOSH's job to digest the data available from the National Cancer Institute, from university scientists, from labor and industry, and elsewhere and recommend to OSHA standards that are adequate to protect workers. It's a mammoth task, but one that is becoming more crucial as the research results and statistics roll in.

NIOSH regards cancer as a special problem, one requiring a new approach to regulation. A major reason is that the tons of unregulated, man-made chemicals being put on the market— more than 700 new chemicals are introduced into industry each year—may be taking their toll in increased cancer rates.

Most known carcinogens in the environment are the direct result of expanding technology in industry and agriculture. Yet, regulation of these chemicals has relied too long on the worker serving as guinea pig. If too many people die, it must mean something needs to be controlled! There is still a wide gap between the strict standards set for health hazards in community air or water and the much more lenient ones set for the workplace.

Increasing agreement among government agencies has persuaded NIOSH that it is time to pay as much attention to the worker as to everyone else. NIOSH uses as its guidelines those principles, agreed upon by various scientific groups, which determine national policy in such areas as regulating chemicals in food. These basic principles, referred to earlier, deserve to be summarized here:

- Any substance that definitely causes tumors in animals should be considered carcinogenic and a potential cancer hazard in man.

- It doesn't matter whether the substance causes benign tumors or malignant ones, since a benign tumor often turns cancerous. There is no chemical known to produce only benign tumors.

- There is no known way to determine a safe level of exposure to any substance known to cause cancer in animals.

These principles have led NIOSH to recommend, and OSHA to adopt, standards of "no detectable exposure" (or its practical equivalent) to such carcinogens as vinyl chloride. NIOSH says an important feature of its policy on carcinogens in the future will be recommendation of a use-permit and registration system for all workplaces where a regulated carcinogen is used. Such a system, the agency believes, will be a giant step toward controlling occupational cancer and will make it easier for scientists to identify plants where a certain chemical has been used.

NIOSH maintains that even suspected carcinogens should be regulated by a permit-registration system. Considering the unknowns, a NIOSH official has said, the agency prefers to err on the side of conservatism when it comes to cancer.

Chapter 9
Controlling Exposure to Carcinogens

TLV? best available technology? ambient level? technological alternatives? What does such government and scientific jargon have to do with protecting workers from cancer?

These confusing terms describe some of the various philosophies for controlling exposure to dangerous substances. The following sections describe how these approaches have been used to limit or eliminate workers' contact with some of the more common job cancer hazards.

Asbestos and the TLV

"Threshold limit value," or TLV, is a term meaning simply the highest level of a substance that a person can be exposed to without suffering certain bad effects. (According to some scientists there is little evidence that thresholds for carcinogens exist; certainly nobody has ever found one.) Generally, the TLV is designed to protect workers from short-term effects—such as irritation or dizziness—brought on by exposure to high concentrations of a chemical. Most of OSHA's current standards are TLVs. But as the case of asbestos demonstrates, the TLV is far from adequate for protecting workers from carcinogens.

Asbestos was one of the first substances for which a TLV was suggested. It also was the target of the first emergency standard and the first permanent standard issued by OSHA under the Occupational Safety and Health Act. Unfortunately, a TLV is probably the least effective way to control exposure to this powerful carcinogen.

The earliest suggestion that a TLV be set for asbestos was made by W. C. Dreessen and several other U.S. Public Health Service scientists in 1938, following a survey of about 500 employees in four North Carolina textile mills. They recommended that asbestos levels be restricted to 5 million particles per cubic foot of air in order to prevent asbestosis—the only disease of concern then. Unfortunately, most of the workers these scientists studied had had only about 10 years' or less exposure to asbestos, so very little was known about the longer term effects.

Nevertheless, this TLV survived as the only guide for controlling asbestos exposure in the United States for more than 30 years. In 1968 it became a legally enforceable standard under the Walsh-Healy Act for those companies doing more than $10,000 worth of business with the federal government. In 1960 the same TLV was adopted as a national asbestos standard in Great Britain.

When it became obvious that workers were still getting asbestosis, both Britain and the United States lowered the number of particles permitted per unit. Shortly after the Occupational Safety and Health Act took effect in 1971, OSHA was pressured by organized labor into issuing a temporary emergency standard and then a final standard of five fibers longer than five micrometers in length per milliliter of air. The limit was to drop to two fibers on July 1, 1976.

Even this standard was based on a British standard, *still designed only to prevent asbestosis.* It wasn't until October 1975, when OSHA proposed a new standard of 0.5 fibers per milliliter and when NIOSH recommended a new standard of 0.1 fibers per milliliter, that lung cancer was mentioned as a concern in controlling asbestos exposure! But even 0.1 fibers per milliliter means 100,000 of these long fibers in each cubic meter of air, and a worker inhales about 8 cubic meters in a working day.

Amid all these efforts to set a threshold limit for asbestos, one fact is clear: no solid evidence exists to suggest that there is such a thing as a safe level for a carcinogen. Therefore, it is impossible, when dealing with carcinogens, to set a true threshold limit value. At any level above zero, there will be *some* risk from asbestos. Standards that allow any exposure, then, are really "risk limitation values." At best, we might reduce the risk by lowering the levels workers may be exposed to.

Studies by Mount Sinai School of Medicine show, however, that although deaths from asbestosis among asbestos workers went down as dustiness decreased, deaths from lung cancer were not necessarily reduced. Those workers who were heavily exposed died from asbestosis before reaching the age when they would be at highest risk of developing lung cancer: lowering their dust exposure kept them alive long enough for some to die of lung cancer or mesothelioma.

Attempting to control asbestos with a TLV also ignores several other thorny problems:

- Asbestos, combined with other substances, especially cigarette smoke, can have a devastating effect. Asbestos workers who smoke have up to 90 times greater risk of dying of lung cancer than do people who neither smoke nor work with asbestos. Figuring the effect of smoking into a standard on asbestos is probably scientifically impossible.

- A TLV does nothing to protect family members who come into contact with dusty clothing, or those people who live near an asbestos plant. They do not benefit from work practices that, in addition to a TLV, might help protect workers inside the plant. Workers might spend their days in conditions that meet official standards, but dust brought home on their clothes could still expose family members to enough asbestos to cause disease.

- Even when the law says that a certain exposure level must be maintained, enforcement of such a standard is shaky at best. OSHA has a jurisdiction of some 5 million workplaces and a meager force of a couple of hundred industrial hygienists to inspect them (data from 1975).

With such a situation, *many* employers are not complying with the law. This was highlighted in a 1972 survey of members of the AFL-CIO's International Association of Heat and Frost

Insulators and Asbestos Workers, conducted by doctors at Mount Sinai. Even though the standard then in effect required that at least one dust count be taken in each workplace where asbestos was used, only 171 of 4,956 workers surveyed had seen a dust count taken where they worked. Of those who had seen counts, 54 worked in shipyards or chemical plants that had permanent industrial hygiene staffs.

The conclusion is that even if we could find an acceptable level of exposure for workers, the government is not now capable of enforcing that level throughout an industry as extensive as the asbestos industry.

So what do we do about asbestos? Ban its use in all forms? Currently, nearly 1 million tons of the mineral are used each year in the United States. For some uses, such as in brake linings, it is difficult at present to find a substitute. Even if asbestos were banned, the country would still face the enormous problems of controlling the large amounts around in some form. Many persons agree that the best solution at the present time is to limit exposure to asbestos and other dangerous, but valuable, substances to the lowest levels possible with existing technology.

Even setting a TLV for these materials can be useful for stimulating development of new engineering controls and for identifying and eliminating those processes that cannot be controlled. To some extent, this has happened in the asbestos industry. Dust conditions are much better in many plants, and asbestos has been eliminated from many insulation products. As improved technology makes lower exposure levels possible, federal standards should, of course, keep pace.

Vinyl chloride—the best available technology

The fatal liver tumor caused by exposure to vinyl chloride —like mesothelioma among asbestos workers—is an example of a rare cancer that would be virtually eliminated if occupational exposure to these substances did not occur, although it would still be necessary to also control exposures associated with end-product use. The truly alarming thing is that with a latency period of 20 years or more, many more of these cancers—the result of past exposures—will show up in years to come.

We can't wait for the body count to rise before we take action to control exposures. Yet, considering the importance of chemical production to all segments of the economy—the worker as well as the employer—the solution cannot be so simple as to eliminate *all* chemicals suspected of causing cancer.

Control, then, of a substance like vinyl chloride must be based on the best available evidence of its effects and the best available technology for preventing worker exposure. Decisions made by OSHA in setting a permanent standard on vinyl chloride have set the stage for future standards on workplace cancer hazards.

Four crucial decisions reached in setting a vinyl chloride standard were:

- A certain level of a substance can be considered to cause cancer in humans even if there is no definite proof that it already has done so.

- It is unwise to assume that humans are less sensitive to vinyl chloride exposure than are laboratory animals if there is no conclusive evidence that this is so.

- All the evidence is not in. Scientists cannot pinpoint the precise level of exposure that poses a hazard or even be sure whether there is a safe level of exposure to vinyl chloride. But as long as workers' lives are at stake, the government cannot wait until these questions are definitely answered. Therefore, OSHA concluded in the preamble to its vinyl chloride standard, "we have had to exercise our best judgment on the basis of the best available evidence. These judgments have required a balancing process, in which the overriding consideration has been the protection of employees, even those who may have regular exposures to vinyl chloride throughout their working lives."

- The required exposure limit of one part of vinyl chloride per million parts of air (ppm), then, is based on the best available evidence and the best available technology.

This decision process clearly reflects the mandate of the Occupational Safety and Health Act, which says that the final decision in controlling job hazards must be that standard ". . . which most adequately assures, to the extent feasible, on the basis of the best available evidence, that no employee will suffer impairment of health or functional capacity even if such employee has regular exposure to the hazard dealt with by such standard for the period of his working life."

Arsenic—keeping it down to the "ambient level"

Some carcinogens, such as arsenic, occur naturally in the environment. This natural level is called the *ambient level*. Obviously, it is impossible to completely prevent exposure to a substance that is present in nature.

But since studies of various groups of workers indicate that arsenic causes cancer in at least three body tissues—skin, lungs, and the lymphatic system—it is important that job exposures not add to the body's natural burden of arsenic. NIOSH has concluded, therefore, that occupational exposures to arsenic should be limited to approximately the ambient level found in the United States.

Benzidine and 2-naphthylamine—voluntary substitution of less dangerous chemicals

Exposure to certain aromatic amines and their derivatives is known to cause bladder cancer among industrial workers. Because the chemical industry usually produces several aromatic amines in the same general area and because workers are exposed to various chemicals as they move from one job to another within a plant, it has been difficult to pin down which compounds are most hazardous.

Nevertheless, there is solid evidence pointing to two aromatic amines—benzidine and 2-naphthylamine—as potent carcinogens in man. A study by Dr. R. A. M. Case of 4,600 British chemical workers revealed 10 times more deaths from bladder cancer than expected among men who had been exposed only to benzidine. More than 80 times as many bladder cancer deaths as expected occurred among workers exposed only to

2-naphthylamine. Beyond the cases recorded as causes of death, numerous other instances of bladder cancer were identified among workers exposed only to these two chemicals.

In the face of this overwhelming evidence, the United Kingdom in 1967 officially prohibited use of known bladder carcinogens. Other aromatic amines suspected of causing cancer were strictly controlled. Workers who might be exposed to them must have medical examinations at least every six months.

The British chemical industry, however, did not wait for official action. After the industry-financed study of chemical workers showed extremely high cancer rates, manufacturers in 1953 followed the lead of industries in some European countries and voluntarily stopped using 2-naphthylamine. The industry was able to substitute other processes or products for each of the important derivatives of this deadly chemical.

The search for benzidine substitutes has been more difficult, and the British chemical industry only recently stopped manufacturing and using benzidine entirely.* In Italy, manufacturers have introduced a number of alternatives to benzidine dyes for use in dyeing cotton. These are somewhat more expensive than the dyes they replace.

Finding adequate substitutes, however, becomes more crucial as evidence mounts that benzidine causes bladder cancer. Adding to the hazard is the textile industry's practice of repeating a dyeing process when cloth does not dye uniformly. This process may release large quantities of aromatic amines.

Probably the most widespread use of benzidine is in the laboratory test for occult blood (the blood in excrement or secretion not clearly evident to the naked eye), and here too, there are promising substitutes that appear to be safer.

The point is that, with advances in modern chemical engineering, many hazardous substances probably could be produced safely, but their *use* in other manufacturing processes is far more difficult to control. The crucial question regarding any occupational carcinogen is whether there are, or will be, any important uses for which no practical substitutes can be found.

* However, see footnote on page 4.

Aldrin and dieldrin—banned!

These two pesticides were judged to pose such a wide-spread cancer hazard that the U.S. Environmental Protection Agency in October 1974 suspended all future production, sale, and use. Studies have shown that these chemicals cause liver cancer in several animal species. In mice, dieldrin causes cancer at the lowest dose yet tested—0.1 parts per million (ppm).

The government acted, though, because the pesticides seriously contaminate our food, air, and water. Surveys indicate that at least a third of all children age five or under, as well as people in other age groups, are getting more than their acceptable daily intake of dieldrin—and the acceptable daily intake was set *before* dieldrin was definitely identified as a carcinogen. Further, dieldrin was found in more than 85 percent of air samples monitored by the government.

This widespread exposure to a hazardous chemical is involuntary and happens without the knowledge or consent of the public. Given the convincing evidence of a hazard, the government concluded that protection of the public health demanded that further production and use of these pesticides be stopped.

This is an excellent example of how the government's standards for safeguarding the general public are much higher than for protecting the worker. Despite the evidence that certain substances are killing many workers, no *workplace* carcinogen has yet been banned in the United States.

Chapter 10
Identifying High-Risk Groups

Identifying and regularly examining workers known to be at high risk of developing occupational cancer can be valuable for learning more about cancer risks, as well as for detecting, and treating, cancer in its early stages.

This chapter describes some of the ways in which scientists are keeping close watch on high-risk groups.

Early warning signs—looking for abnormal cells

Through microscope examination of cells from body tissues —such as the respiratory and urinary tracts—doctors can detect cancer in its very early stages, before it spreads, and while chances for successful treatment *may* still be good. Such tests also provide a good picture of the risk faced by workers exposed to certain substances.

Italian scientists, for example, have found a high incidence of abnormal cells in the respiratory tracts of workers exposed to chromium pigments and vinyl chloride and among chemical workers in general. The rate of abnormalities was even higher than that among heavy smokers who did not work in the chemical industry.

Similarly, they found a surprisingly high rate of abnormal cells in the urine of 470 workers from four dyestuff factories who were exposed to aromatic amines. These workers are known to be at high risk of developing bladder cancer.

Such tests can be both more effective and less hazardous than x-rays for regular health monitoring. Some studies have shown that repeated x-rays may increase susceptibility to leukemia—a side effect that can be especially dangerous for people already at high risk of developing cancer.

Then too, by the time a cancer, particularly lung cancer, is detectable by x-ray, it is usually too late for treatment to prolong the victim's life. "When you institute screening methods, you should make sure that you're not only detecting tumors, but also prolonging survival," says Dr. Lorne Houten of Roswell Park Memorial Institute in Buffalo, N.Y. "Otherwise, you're just giving the poor patient more years to worry about his tumor."

Sputum cytology—analysis of respiratory tract cells contained in a sample of coughed-up sputum—has been a routine procedure for more than 20 years. It is now believed by some doctors to be a valuable method for detecting lung cancer long before the disease shows up on x-rays and has given scientists a clearer picture of how lung cancer develops.

Regular sputum cytology tests of some 3,000 uranium workers since 1957 have shown that it takes an average of about four years for a lung cancer to develop from the stage where abnormal cells can be detected to where the cancer has become invasive. As the disease progresses, cells in the lung become more and more obviously abnormal to the trained eye until what is called an *in situ*, or localized, cancer develops. In this stage, large numbers of malignant cells can be identified in the sputum. This prompt detection, followed by surgery, holds promise for increasing lung cancer survival rates.

Doctors at the Ministry of Health in Toronto, Canada, have had good success with sputum monitoring of nickel plant workers who run a high risk of lung cancer because of exposure to a heat-treatment process that releases carcinogens from the ore. After enlisting the cooperation of labor unions and carefully explaining details to workers themselves, the Ministry of Health launched a cytology monitoring program among nickel workers in the Sudbury district of Ontario, the area that is the world's greatest single source of nickel.

These doctors reported that of the 282 men examined in 1973 and 1974, abnormal cells were identified in 11. Of those, 10 had no x-ray evidence of disease and no significant symptoms. Several have since had successful surgery to remove localized cancers detected by the cytology tests.

The directors of this project are enthusiastic about further early detection and successful treatment. They point to the success rate at Toronto General Hospital, where since 1960 doctors have performed surgery in 22 cases of lung cancer that were detected by cytology tests but invisible on x-rays. One patient died in surgery; the other 21 are still alive three to 15 years after surgery.

In this country, perhaps the best known cancer monitoring effort is the Tyler Asbestos Workers Program, designed to provide early detection and treatment of disease among nearly 900 former employees of a Tyler, Texas, asbestos plant that was in operation from 1954 to 1972. Approximately 90 percent of the former workers are cigarette smokers, and this history plus their past exposure to asbestos makes them extremely likely to develop lung cancer.

Under a contract from the National Cancer Institute, doctors from the Texas Chest Foundation, East Texas Chest Hospital, and Baylor College of Medicine examine each worker every six months. The men undergo a complete physical examination and a battery of tests—including a chest x-ray, measurement of breathing capacity, and analysis of a sputum sample.

Looking at job histories—and hobbies

A study at Roswell Park Memorial Institute in Buffalo, N.Y., has shown that hospital records can help scientists identify certain occupational groups at high risk of cancer. Unfortunately, many hospital records are woefully lacking in information about the patient's work history. Researchers stress that every questionnaire used by doctors and hospitals should include information about jobs and hobbies—which, incidentally, can also be a source of exposure to carcinogens.

If a person avidly pursues a hobby such as painting or

photography, his exposure to hazardous chemicals could be similar to that of an industrial worker. Dr. Rulon Rawson of the University of Texas System Cancer Center tells of a patient whose bone marrow indicated previous exposure to humata-toxins. The patient reported that he had used large amounts of a paint remover containing benzol. "When I told his physician I thought his disease was related to benzol exposure, the response was, 'Can't be. He's a policeman.' My response was, 'Only for 40 hours a week.' "

Obviously, in looking for environmental carcinogens we should look for them not only in the workplace, but in the home and other places where an individual might pursue his hobbies.

Mapping cancer rates

A National Cancer Institute study charting cancer death rates in individual counties of the United States strongly suggests a link between high cancer rates and exposure to industrial pollutants—especially in the Northeast and in the urban areas around the Great Lakes. Researchers simply charted death rates from various types of cancer in specific counties and then found out what kinds of industries employ the most people in those areas.

The study showed consistently high death rates from lung cancer along the Gulf Coast from Texas through Florida, with the heaviest concentration in Louisiana. High rates also were found along the south Atlantic coast and in northern New Jersey, New York City, and along the Hudson River. These areas have almost twice the national proportion of people working in manufacturing of chemicals and allied products and twice the proportion making paper and allied products.

It is "nearly certain," the Cancer Institute says, that on-the-job exposures were responsible for the striking concentration of bladder cancer deaths among men in the East. The highest bladder cancer rate in the country was in Salem County, N.J., where 25 percent of the population works in chemical plants. One company in the area has reported that at least 330 workers from a single plant have developed bladder cancer over the past 50 years.

Aside from New Jersey, bladder cancer was concentrated in urban areas around the Great Lakes and in rural New York and New England. These areas have large numbers of people working in the manufacture of professional scientific and control instruments; lumber and wood products; chemicals and allied products; and stone, clay, and glass products.

Scientists suspect that high bladder cancer rates in rural areas with sawmills and planing mills may be related to earlier findings of nasal and sinus cancer among wood-workers in the furniture industry. Both nasal cancer and bladder cancer also have been found among shoe and leather workers. Among these groups, it appears that a carcinogen is acting both at the site of intake (the nose) and the site of excretion (the urinary tract).

The cancer map also shows cases of kidney cancer clustered in rural Wisconsin, Minnesota, and the Dakotas. These areas have concentrations of petroleum refining and lumber and wood products industries.

The Cancer Institute cautions that there are several limitations to these findings: the researchers did not know the occupations of the people who died from cancer; there was no way to consider the impact of smoking; and there may have been regional variations in the diagnosis of disease.

However, the study does show how geographical patterns of cancer may help identify carcinogens in the workplace. Although it isn't practical to investigate every industry in the United States for cancer hazards, it is possible to chart the kinds of industries located in those areas with high cancer rates. Any leads that develop from such a map can then be pursued through more detailed studies of death records and surveys of workers in those areas.

Part IV
A "SOCIAL DISEASE"

More than 700 new chemicals are introduced into industry each year. At the same time, we are discovering that a large proportion of all human cancers are due to environmental agents, including chemicals. For the "chemical tumors," the majority are caused by chemicals man himself has introduced into the environment.

We have to ask ourselves, as a society, some tough questions: Are convenience plastics, or certain shades of dyes, or other chemical wonders worth the price in workers' health? Or, for that matter, the general public's health?

The real issue in occupational cancer is not so much *if* we can prevent it as whether we are *willing* to prevent it. Occupational cancer is a "social disease," a disease whose causes and control are deeply rooted in the technology and economy of our society. Prevention of cancer is largely an attainable goal, but it requires the coordinated effort of all parts of society: government, the scientific community, industry, labor, and an informed public.

Chapter 11
The Risky Business of Determining Risk

When scientists or economists or politicians talk about "risk assessment," they mean the process of figuring out the probability that bad results will occur under a specific set of circumstances. In occupational health, risk assessment comes down to a matter of whether the social or economic value of a certain chemical is great enough to justify the risk to workers' health or lives.

Too often scientists and government experts discuss risk in terms of whether or not there is a safe level of exposure to a carcinogen or what is a minimal acceptable level of exposure, when the real problem is that thousands of people continue to be exposed to large, uncontrolled amounts of cancer-causing substances every day.

Unfortunately, determining the level of risk associated with use of a chemical is often haphazard. Not all scientists agree with the results of animal tests or studies of specific groups of workers. There is always some question about how well we can determine what a small dose of a chemical will do to a human being by studying what a large dose does to a rat.

Studies also are hampered by inadequate records of workers' medical and job histories. Few workers spend a lifetime in the same job, and even if they do, it's unlikely that they are exposed throughout their work lives to the same level of the same substances. Many workers—mechanics or pipefitters, for example—work anywhere in a plant and are exposed to countless hazards.

In the past, industry has not readily revealed information about the hazards in its factories. As Sheldon Samuels of the AFL-CIO's Industrial Union Department points out, many decent people in management actually don't know that hazards exist because they have hired as medical directors or consultants "yes-men" who tell them what it is thought they want to hear about working conditions. Worse yet, most major corporations in the country have made conscious decisions not even to hire full-time medical directors.

The government is guilty of foot-dragging in setting standards on dangerous workplace chemicals. There are at least several dozen compounds that definitely cause cancer in animals for which no federal standards have yet been issued. Too often it seems that the government simply is unwilling to put workers' health above political and economic considerations.

Workers themselves have long been kept in the dark about what they work with and what those substances can do to them. This lack of information prevents them from making crucial judgments about the risks they face just by going to work every day.

The difficulty in determining risk, then, is not just scientific. As Sheldon Samuels bluntly puts it, the matter of risk in occupational health ". . . comes down to the question of who shall live and who shall die. We simply cannot continue to build industries around unscreened toxic substances."

Chapter 12
Protection vs. Profits

It's hard to believe that money could be an issue when it comes to protecting people from cancer. Yet, a favorite argument against stricter health standards is that they would be inflationary. The increased cost to industry of complying with new standards would boost the cost of products, the argument goes, and that cost would be passed on to consumers, adding to the inflationary spiral.

Such short-sighted logic focuses only on the immediate costs of new standards and ignores the long-term benefits— especially prevention of cancer among certain groups of workers two or three decades from now. It also ignores the fact that disease, health care, and environmental damage are costly, even though these costs cannot be as easily indexed as a 15 percent increase in the market price of a product.

Dr. Paul Kotin, vice-president for medical affairs at Johns Manville Corporation, has calculated that environmentally caused diseases cost the nation some $35 billion a year. Our society tolerates this burden because it is hidden in ever-increasing costs for medical attention of all kinds. What we must recognize is that this crushing cost will rise even more if we continue to deal with occupational and environmental diseases after the fact instead of preventing them in the first place.

Industry argues that withdrawing from the market a chemical that has been produced in large amounts would be an economic disaster and that reshaping a manufacturing process in order to protect workers would increase production costs to impossible levels. Persons who put forth these arguments forget the profits already made from production of a hazardous chemical.

The government itself has delayed badly needed OSHA standards on such carcinogens as arsenic and coke-oven emissions by requiring "economic impact statements." According to organized labor, these documents, outlining the costs and benefits of new standards, are simply political devices and are illegal because they are mentioned nowhere in the Occupational Safety and Health Act.

An example of government's placing economic considerations ahead of workers' lives came during June 1972 when George Guenther, then Assistant Secretary for OSHA, wrote to an official in the Department of Labor that during the next four years ". . . no highly controversial standards will be proposed by OSHA or NIOSH." Unfortunately for the nation's workers, some people claim, OSHA kept its promise.

In all the talk about costs, the individual worker and his family are rarely considered. Yet they are the ones who pay the real price with their suffering.

Take the case of a worker who developed asbestosis (and has since died) while working for Pittsburgh Corning in Port Allegheny, Pa. He was forced to accept $36 a week in compensation, supplemented by community welfare funds. He and his fellow workers had been told by company doctors that they were not exposed to any dangerous substances.

What does $36 a week mean? Obviously, it means the impoverishment of an entire family. It means that the priority in medical care is not prolonging a man's life but simply easing his painful death. As Sheldon Samuels of the AFL-CIO points out, that man no longer had the lung capacity even to say the words "corporate responsibility."

B.F. Goodrich, which reaped much favorable publicity for voluntarily breaking the news about vinyl chloride in 1974, began paying compensation as long ago as 1965 to workers afflicted with vinyl chloride disease. The first victim died of angiosarcoma, the rare liver cancer now known to be caused by exposure to vinyl chloride. Yet, as far as is known, the company did little to clean up the plant. In fact, the workers lost a strike in which one of the demands was for an eating place free of polyvinyl chloride dust and vinyl chloride fumes.

This attitude is especially unhappy in light of evidence that improvements in manufacturing processes—which usually mean just a marginal loss of profit instead of a severe blow to the economy of a plant—can drastically reduce exposures to hazardous substances and decrease the incidence of disease among workers. Nickel workers in the United Kingdom and Norway, for example, who started working after an industrial process had been modified, do not have the high rates of nasal sinus and lung cancer found among earlier nickel workers.

Chapter 13
The Worker's Right to Know

It seems only logical that those most affected by hazardous substances—the people who work with them—should be rapidly informed about the danger. By granting workers the right to a safe workplace, the Occupational Safety and Health Act mandates that workers have the right to know when and if they are exposed to carcinogens and what is being done to protect them. Workers also have the right to know that scientists, with their present knowledge about cancer, cannot say that any particular exposure to a carcinogen is absolutely safe; there are no "guarantees."

Yet, as most workers will attest, it's a long way from having the right to know and actually knowing. Information about who is at risk from what has long been the domain of academic, industrial, and government scientists—and even some union leaders. In many cases, for a variety of reasons, they waited for long periods before sharing their information with workers.

Knowledge is crucial if workers are going to have any say in their own protection. They need scientific information so that they can participate in the standards-setting process and make sure that any new standard has adequate provisions for medical examinations and regular monitoring of the workplace. And once a standard is set, informed workers can ensure that it is properly enforced in their plants.

If there is no federal standard, or if the standard in effect doesn't recognize that a substance may cause cancer, there is an even greater need for workers to be informed so they can take steps—through collective bargaining or "friendly persuasion"—to protect themselves until the government sets an adequate standard.

Instead, workers have generally been denied the most basic information: which substances cause cancer or even what chemicals they are working with. *Even workers who are informed about carcinogens cannot take action to protect themselves if they don't know the ingredients behind the trade names of the chemicals they work with.*

The issue of the worker's right to know was the basis of two recent cases brought to arbitration by the Oil, Chemical, and Atomic Workers' Union. In the first case, workers at a Ciba-Geigy agricultural products plant in McIntosh, Alabama, knew that some of the chemicals they worked with were dangerous and asked for a list of all chemicals they were exposed to. The company balked at this request, and after filing of grievances, the case went to arbitration.

In the second case, workers at an Arco polymers plant near Pittsburgh knew the names of most of the chemicals they worked with and were aware that at least one was dangerous, because from time to time the company took blood tests to check for ill effects. However, when the workers wanted a physician other than the company doctor to take a look at the results to see how severe the health hazard was, the company refused.

What the workers at Arco didn't know then was that the "dangerous" chemical was benzene—a solvent that some 2 million American workers are exposed to, and to which *at least* 150 documented cases of leukemia in workers around the world are attributed. The Arco employees knew only that every so often the company doctor said a worker had to be transferred to another part of the plant until his white blood cell count returned to normal. They had no idea that benzene was suspected of causing cancer or how serious a risk they were running by working with this chemical.

The union argued before federal arbitration judges that

workers could not participate meaningfully in collective bargaining, which involves assessing job health risks, without knowledge of the chemicals they worked with or the effects of those chemicals on their health. In both cases, the judge ruled in favor of the workers, establishing at last the worker's right to know—a victory long in coming. It is to be hoped that other workers throughout the country will soon hear of these decisions.

Workers are often uninformed about the role of smoking in occupational cancer. Despite all the antismoking hullabaloo in the media, few workers have been told point blank that they absolutely should not smoke. Neither industry nor government has informed workers that smoking, on top of exposure even to weak carcinogens on the job, increases their risk of developing cancer. This surely is basic information the worker needs in order to determine just how dangerous a position he/she is in.

Everybody's got an excuse for neglecting to inform the worker. Industry officials say they don't want to tell workers about evidence that certain substances cause cancer in animals because they are "afraid of scaring them."

Scientists are naturally cautious people who prefer to wait until all the evidence is in before they make any "final" conclusions. Unfortunately, additional evidence often comes in the form of a higher body count. Workers continue to die without even knowing they were in danger and without any protection from standards that were delayed because "all the evidence wasn't in."

All workers have the right to know, especially when the subject is cancer. Scientists and industry and government officials have the moral responsibility to share with workers whatever knowledge they have, even if it is limited at this time.

This book is a step in that direction. It is a tool for seeking a safer workplace. Use it.